Health Benefits of Turmeric - Curcumin

For Cooking and Health

By M. Usman

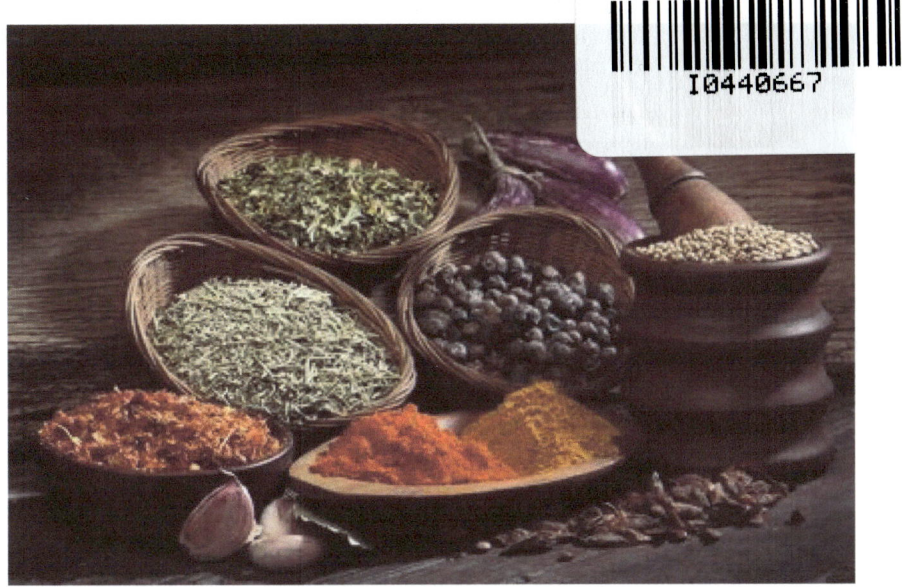

Health Learning Series

Mendon Cottage Books

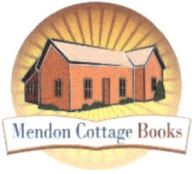

JD-Biz Publishing

Download Free Books!

http://MendonCottageBooks.com

Disclaimer

The information is this book is provided for informational purposes only. It is not intended to be used and medical advice or a substitute for proper medical treatment by a qualified health care provider. The information is believed to be accurate as presented based on research by the author.

The contents have not been evaluated by the U.S. Food and Drug Administration or any other Government or Health Organization and the contents in this book are not to be used to treat cure or prevent disease or mental illness.

The author or publisher is not responsible for the use or safety of any diet, procedure or treatment mentioned in this book. The author or publisher is not responsible for errors or omissions that may exist.

Warning

The Book is for informational purposes only and before taking on any diet, treatment or medical procedure it is recommended to consult with your primary care provider.

Our books are available at

1. Amazon.com
2. Barnes and Noble
3. Itunes
4. Kobo
5. Smashwords
6. Google Play Books

Table of Contents

Preface

Nature has given us cures to every disease known to man in one form or another yet we still choose to pick synthetic treatments full of side-effects over them. These cures are right in front of us but we fail to see them; turmeric is one of these cures hidden in plain sight.

Everyone in the western world knows turmeric when it comes to making curries but it is probably the most underestimated and least popular spice when it comes to its medicinal uses. For starters, turmeric is a plant from which the spice of the same name is obtained. The most common form of turmeric is its powder form, which is of bright yellow color. The use of turmeric for flavoring, for cosmetic purposes and for medicinal uses goes back to the Vedic period in India and it is since then that it has had a massive impact over the region which explains its high demand in most Indian households.

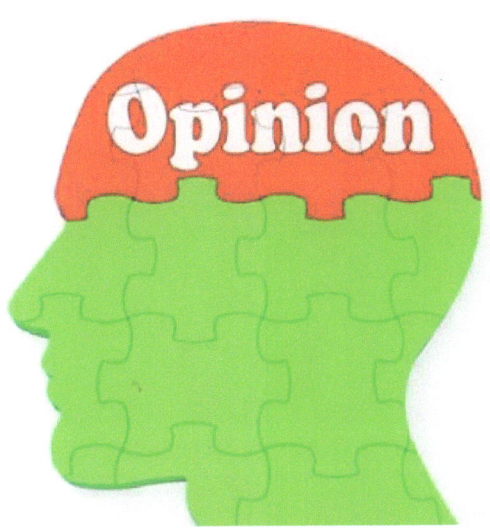

This book will tell you about the health benefits of turmeric and how it cures & help fight fatal ailments. After reading this book, you will be surprised about how little you knew about this super spice and how including it in your daily life can bring back your body from the verge of expiration.

Getting Started

Chapter # 1: Intro

The history of turmeric can be traced as back as 3000BC when it was native only to Indonesia and Southern India. Turmeric was of such importance that it found its way into traditional Indian medicine called the Ayurveda.

As mentioned previously turmeric is basically a plant and its real name is Curcuma longa, belonging to the ginger family, Zingiberaceae. The spice turmeric is obtained from the roots of the plant, which have tough brown skin and a deep orange flesh when peeled. It is from this flesh that the powder obtains its characteristic color. Turmeric powder has a warm, peppery yet bitter taste with a slight fragrance of a mixture of orange and ginger.

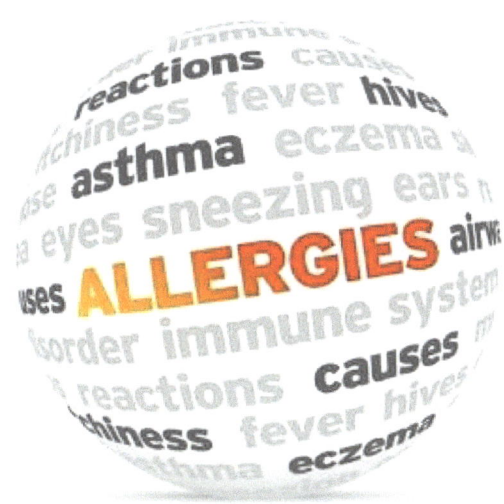

Animal and laboratory studies have found out that turmeric possess a chemical that has anti-oxidant along with cancer inhibiting properties. Other health benefits of turmeric include relief from arthritis, diarrhea, bloating and conditions affecting the liver. Though to be specific turmeric can offer protection against bronchitis, headaches, common cold, leprosy, fever, menstrual problems, depression, Alzheimer and kidney complications.

But the list of benefits does not end here and keeps on going; from being a pesticide to a food preserver to a flavoring agent, turmeric has played a vital role in traditions and customs of the Eastern world that are just, now being availed by the other half of the world.

Chapter # 2: Nutritional Facts

The power that turmeric packs is enormous; just a few grams of turmeric a day in any form, be it powder, fresh or crushed root, can provide ample nutrients to keep diseases like anemia, memory dysfunctions and neuritis at bay.

The following chart shows the nutritional facts of a 2tbsp (4.40g) serving of turmeric.

Basic Macronutrient and Calories	
Nutrient	**Amount**
Protein	0.34g
Carbohydrates	2.86g
Fat- total	0.43g
Dietary Fiber	0.93g
Calories	15.58

The following chart shows the minerals contained in a 2tbsp (4.40g) serving of turmeric.

Minerals	
Nutrient	**Amount**
Calcium	8.05mg
Copper	0.03mg
Iron	1.82mg
Magnesium	8.49mg

Manganese	0.34mg
Phosphorus	11.79mg
Potassium	111.10mg
Selenium	0.20mcg
Sodium	1.67mg
Zinc	0.19mg

Of all the minerals and nutrients listed, magnesium, iron and fatty acids stand out to be the most vital minerals for the body and are responsible for various key functions in the human body that keeps it stable. The importance of these minerals to the human body is explained below:

1.   Magnesium:

Magnesium is responsible for over 300 biochemical functions in the human body. These functions vary from keeping the heart's rhythm stable to supporting the immune system to keeping the bones strengthened. So if you're running low on magnesium, sprinkle turmeric over magnesium rich products like broccoli, black beans, tofu, spinach, peanuts, almonds and pumpkin seeds.

2.   Iron:

Only a single teaspoon of turmeric powder can charge your body's iron requirements by 16 percent. Iron is so vital for your body that without it, your body's red blood cells will decrease which would cause severe weakness and fatigue. Combining turmeric with spices rich in iron can be one way of getting rid of this deficiency; these spices include coriander, garlic and celery seeds. Otherwise, you can sprinkle turmeric on lean meats, leafy vegetables and clams to keep your body's iron to a healthy level.

3. Fatty Acids:

In a single teaspoon of turmeric powder lay more than 32mg of omega-3 and 114mg of omega-6 fatty acids. These fatty acids are responsible for enhancing cognitive ability, keeping arteries clear and reducing inflammation. Therefore, remember to add a few teaspoons of turmeric to salmon or turkey to keep your fatty acid reserves up to the mark.

Chapter # 3: Uses of Turmeric

Apart from its medicinal properties turmeric finds it use in almost others aspects of human lives that include:

• Due to its unique color and rich flavor turmeric is used in curries and gravies of all kind.

• It is increasingly being used as a preservative. Researchers in India have concluded that turmeric powder can be used to preserve cottage cheese and extend its shelf life by 12 days.

• Mixing turmeric powder with water can give you a household pesticide; sprinkling this over any entry point of your house can ward off ants, insects and termites.

• Turmeric finds its use in dermatologist recommended skin products such as body scrubs. In fact this particular use of turmeric has been capitalized by Indians for centuries at their weddings to give the bride a golden glow.

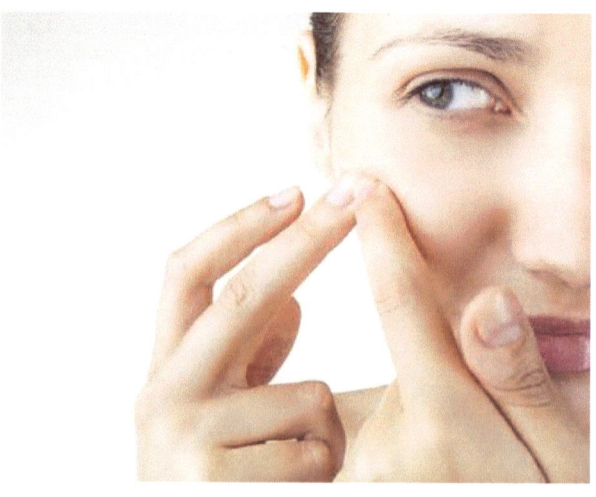

- Former beauty queen Susie Castillo has revealed that she used her own homemade toothpaste that contained turmeric to whiten her teeth. This may come as a surprise to many people due to the color of turmeric but turmeric does work as a teeth whitener given the fact that it does not remain in contact with the teeth for over 30 minutes.

- Turmeric is also used as dye in south-east Asian countries. Furthermore, in combination with annatto, another plant, turmeric is used to color yogurt, cheese, margarine, salad, mustards and canned chicken broths.

Chapter # 4: Storing Turmeric

Nowadays, dry herbs and spices are easily available from any grocery store or supermarkets but still it is preferable if you explore you area for local spice dealers and ethnic markets. These stores may not attract you in the same way that big, departmental chains do but the quality as well as variety of herbs & spices you can find in these markets is unmatched. When you are picking out turmeric try to choose originally grown turmeric rhizomes, i.e. roots of turmeric plant. The roots of the turmeric plant are chosen as they are less likely to be irradiated and thus, more pure than crushed turmeric.

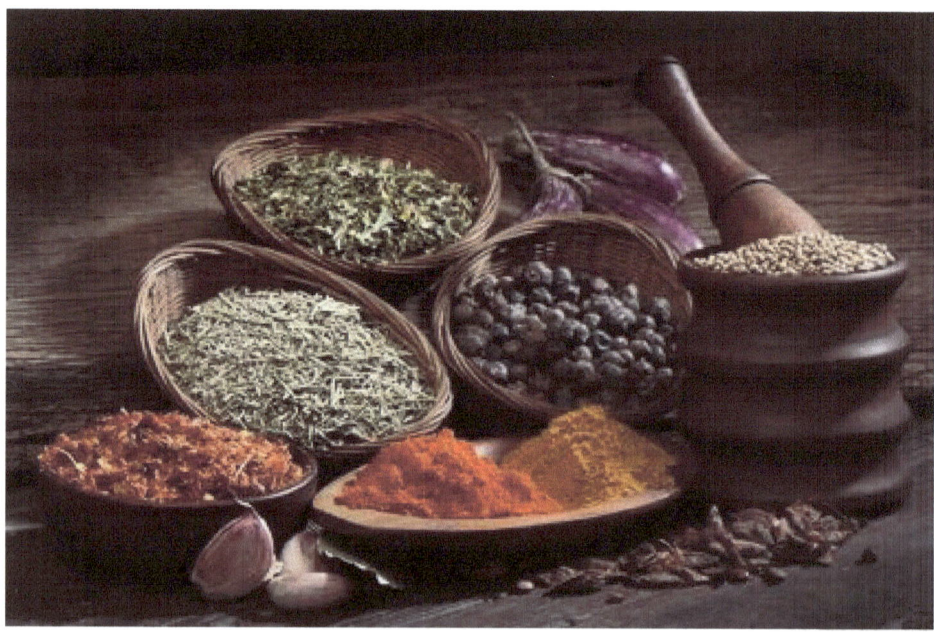

After you have obtained the turmeric rhizomes, you can make your own powder by first boiling, then drying and finally grinding it to the desired level. Remember to store raw rhizomes in a refrigerated environment. This powder should then be kept in cool, dark and dry place in a tightly sealed environment.

If you still choose to buy turmeric from the supermarket, than make sure that you buy turmeric powder rather than curry powder. The true flavor of turmeric is obtained from curcumin. Turmeric contains the highest amount of curcumin when compared to other spices so always choose turmeric powder as it will give you a higher taste and aroma than any other spice.

Chapter #5: Recipes

Eggless Egg Salad

Ingredients:

1. 2 tablespoons mayonnaise
2. 1 tablespoon sweet pickle relish
3. 1 teaspoon distilled white vinegar
4. 1 teaspoon prepared mustard
5. 1 teaspoon white sugar
6. 1/2 teaspoon ground turmeric
7. 1/4 teaspoon dried dill weed
8. 1 tablespoon dried parsley
9. 1 pound firm tofu, sliced and well drained
10. 1 tablespoon minced onion
11. 2 tablespoons minced celery
12. Salt to taste
13. Ground black pepper to taste

Directions:

1. In a small bowl mix mayonnaise, vinegar, sweet pickle relish, sugar, mustard, turmeric, parsley and dill.

2. Place dried tofu in a bowl and crumble it with a fork. Add onion and celery and mix it in the mixture made earlier.

3. Add salt and pepper as per requirement and allow it to chill for several hours so the flavors can blend in.

Sprouted Lentil Veggie Burger

Ingredients:

1. 2 cups sprouted lentils
2. 1 cooked, mashed sweet potato
3. 2 tablespoons butter
4. 3 tablespoons ground flax
5. 1 teaspoon turmeric
6. 2 cloves
7. 1 teaspoon salt
8. 1 teaspoon pepper

Directions:

1. Before starting to make this burger, make sure you have sprouted red lentils.

2. Cook the sweet potatoes in a 400 degrees oven, remove their skin and mash them.

3. Combine the ingredients in a food processor and mix them.

4. Form the mix into patties and cook them in a skillet using butter or oil. After the one half has browned, flip and cook the other half.

5. Serve with avocado, cheese or any other of your favorite toppings.

Orange Turmeric Cake

Ingredients:

1. 250 grams butter
2. 250 grams sugar
3. 4 eggs
4. 150 grams Greek yogurt
5. 20 grams turmeric powder
6. 200 grams almond meal
7. 150 grams polenta
8. 1 teaspoon baking (bicarb) soda
9. 2 oranges
10. ½ cup of thick Greek yogurt
11. ½ cup icing sugar
12. Orange zest to garnish

Directions:

1. Pre-heat your oven to 180 degrees Celsius.
2. Line a 20cm, circular baking tin with baking paper, apply butter to it and coat it with polenta. In a mixing bowl, cream the sugar and butter till it turns pale. Add one egg at a time and mix it till it combines; add and stir the turmeric and yogurt.
3. Add the almond meal, baking (bicarb) soda and polenta and mix them. Then add the zest and juice from the oranges and stir them together.
4. Bake in an oven for 1 hour. After five minutes of cooling turn out the cake. Allow the cake to cool for an hour before icing it.
5. Combine the icing sugar & yogurt and spread it over the top of the cake.

Quick Curried Beef

Ingredients:

1. 1, 3 and a half ounce bag long grain rice
2. 1 pound flank trimmed steak
3. Cooking spray
4. ½ cup sliced onions
5. 1 teaspoon bottled minced garlic
6. 1 tablespoon ground coriander
7. 1 teaspoon ground cumin
8. ½ teaspoon salt
9. ¼ teaspoon ground turmeric
10. 1 can diced tomatoes

Directions:

1. Boil rice according to instructions on the packet.
2. As the rice cook, cut the steak diagonally into thin slices.
3. Coat a large skillet with cooking spray and heat it over medium-high intensity heat. Add garlic and onions and sauté for 2 minutes.
4. Add coriander, salt, cumin and turmeric and sauté for 1 minute.
5. Add steak and sauté for 6 minutes until done.
6. Add tomatoes and reduce the heat intensity to low.
7. Cook for three minutes.
8. Serve with rice.

Beef Curry

Ingredients:

1. 3 tablespoons cooking oil
2. 1 onion
3. 3 cloves
4. 1 tablespoon fresh ginger
5. 2 and a half teaspoons ground coriander
6. 1 teaspoon cumin
7. ¼ teaspoon red-pepper flakes
8. 1/8 teaspoon turmeric
9. ½ tablespoons salt
10. 2 tablespoons water
11. 1 and a half pounds sirloin steak
12. 3 tablespoons chopped cilantro

Directions:

1. In a frying pan, heat the cooking oil over medium heat. Cut the onion into thin slices, add them to the pan and cook until translucent. Add the ginger & garlic and cook for a minute.

2. In a small bowl, combine the cumin, coriander, red-pepper flakes, salt, turmeric and water. Make a paste and cook for a minute while stirring.

3. Cut the steak into 1 inch cubes and cook for 3 minutes. Raise the heat from moderate to high and cook to your liking. If you want medium rare, cook for 5 minutes.

Tagine of Lamb &Apricots in Honey Sauce

Ingredients:

1. 1 teaspoon salt
2. 1 teaspoon ground turmeric
3. ¾ teaspoon ground cinnamon
4. ¼ teaspoon black pepper
5. 2 pounds lamb stew meat
6. 2 teaspoons olive oil
7. 2 cups chopped onion
8. 1 cup beef broth
9. ¼ cup honey
10. 1 cinnamon stick
11. 1 cup dried chopped apricots
12. ¼ cup slivered almonds

Directions:

1. Preheat oven to 425 degrees.

2. Combine ingredients 1-5 in a bowl. Heat oil over medium-high intensity heat and add the contents of the bowl into it. Cook for 5 minutes till all sides of the lamb are brown. Add onion and cook for 2 minutes.

3. Add honey, broth and cinnamon stick. Cover the mixture and bake for 45 minutes in the over.

4. Add apricots and bake another 15 minutes.

Health Benefits of Turmeric

Chapter #6: Introduction

Turmeric has a wide range of health benefits and the principal component to which all these benefits are owed is curcumin. What is curcumin? Curcumin can be defined as a pigment that gives turmeric its brownish-orange color. Currently, curcumin is mostly being used for food coloring but increasing amounts of experiments & studies are proving that curcumin is highly therapeutic; in fact curcumin is already a part of many of the anti-oxidant and anti-inflammatory drugs in the market. The color of curcumin can be found under the food color code E100.

In the subsequent chapters you will find out about the various health benefits of turmeric.

Chapter # 7: Inflammation and Oxidation

Turmeric is a very powerful anti-oxidant and anti-inflammatory agent. It neutralizes free radicals that would otherwise travel through one's body and cause damage to healthy cells and DNA; these oxidants are responsible for chronic conditions like cancer and atherosclerosis. Nowadays, these conditions are on the rise and every artificial treatment in the market costs both money and side-effects but turmeric provides a fully potent and safe, natural anti-inflammatory solution to these conditions.

Turmeric regulates specific inflammatory factors such as enzymes and compounds that hinder the development of these conditions. Combine this with inexpensiveness and no toxic side-effects like ulcer formation, and you get yourself a spice that works like a perfect drug.

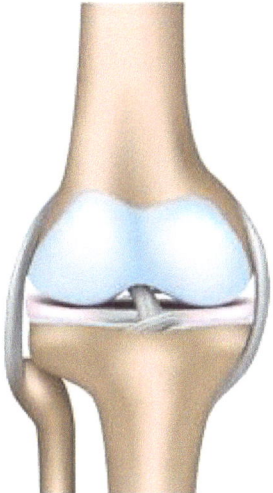 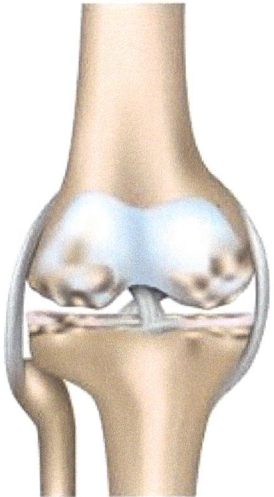

Healthy knee joint   Osteoarthritis

Free-radicals are also responsible for the painful joint inflammation called arthritis which eventually leads to complete deformation of joints. As turmeric is an anti-oxidant it helps deal with this condition too; the simplest example of it working is the relief that an arthritis patient feels after having a warm bowl of spicy soup. A study conducted by the journal *Oncagene* compared the effectiveness of turmeric with phenylbutazone, a synthetic drug used to treat arthritis. It was found out that turmeric was much more helpful as it shortened the duration of stiffness of the joints, especially in the morning; furthermore it lengthened the walking time and reduced the intensity of joint swelling. With all that said, it had no side-effects and therefore, it wouldn't hurt you to consume turmeric rich foods, just to be on the safe side.

Also, when it comes to inflammatory bowel disease, turmeric is proving to be a ground breaking treatment in experiments. Currently, this process is in testing phase but future prospects are bright; experiments carried out on mice have shown that the fraction of mice that were given doses of turmeric were immune to inflammatory agents that induce colitis; moreover they lost less weigh and their intestinal flow was also not affected. This showed that curcumin not only prevented inflammatory diseases but also inhibited a major, cellular inflammatory agent. Human trials are still to be carried out but this technique has been in wide use in South-east Asia for centuries so there is no harm in trying a plate of curry with your favorite rice every alternate evening.

Chapter # 8: Cystic Fibrosis

Cystic Fibrosis is an inherited blood disease caused by one of the most common genetic defects, which unfortunately result in death. Sufferers of cystic fibrosis have their organs blocked by salty, thick mucus that results in life-threatening infections; it affects approximately 30,000 American children and adults, who survive rarely beyond the age of 30.

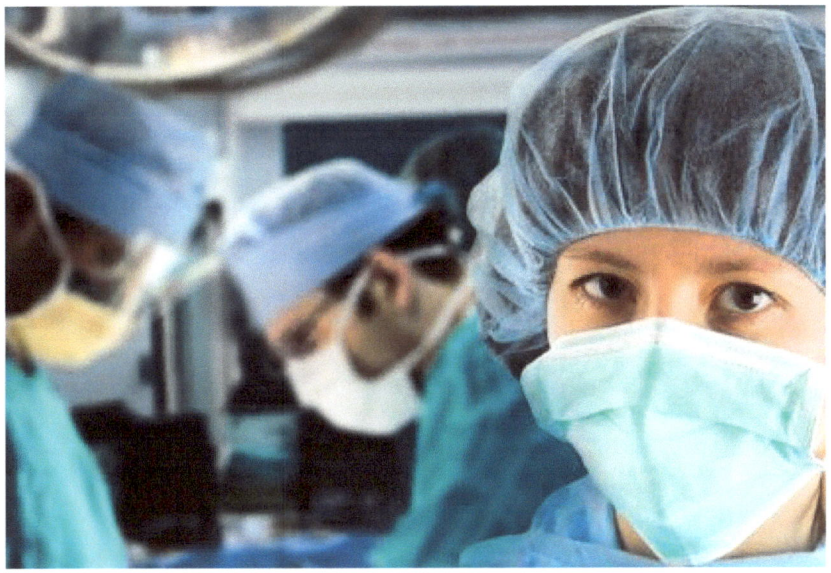

The major symptoms of cystic fibrosis are lung infections, salty sweat and bowel difficulties. The organs at risk include the lungs, pancreas, intestines and the sex organs. In patients of CF, thick and sticky mucus deposits in the lung and prevents correct air flow; this allows bacteria to flourish resulting in infections as stated previously. In the same way it deposits in the pancreas and blocks its ducts; this ceases the flow of enzymes to the small intestine that further causes the food to break down irregularly and incompletely.

One potential weapon against cystic fibrosis is turmeric. Medical explorers at both the University of Washington and John Hopkins University are conducting experiments involving turmeric as a possible agent against cystic fibrosis. The most common gene mutation that causes CF is known as DeltaF508; when mice with this defect were given doses of curcumin, equivalent to human doses; it was found out that this defect was corrected.

When it comes to human trials, a study conducted by Yale researchers has shown that curcumin inhibited the release of calcium which resulted in easy escape of mutated cells that in turn resulted in lower build-up of the salty mucus. Still you should not fall for the quick treatment and take curcumin supplements; instead you should consume turmeric rich foods and you will see significant decrease in saltiness of your sweat. This will be a direct indicator that the turmeric is working!

Chapter # 9: Childhood Leukemia

Leukemia is the cancer of blood cells that originates from the bone marrow. In its normal state, the bone marrow makes white blood that help the body fight numerous infections but under leukemia the body makes defected white blood cells that do nothing except crowding the normal blood cells. This leads to problems such as infections from wounds, bleeding and anemia.

The risk of childhood leukemia has suddenly increased especially after the 20th century; since the 1950s the risk of a child under the age of five, developing leukemia has increased by 50%. The exact reason is still not known but the urban environmental factors and life-style are thought to be the major players in this area. One strange thing though is that this condition is much lower in Asian countries than most Western nations.

Professor Moolky Nagabhushan of the Loyala University Medical Centre, Chicago has conducted studies over the last 20 years to find a solid answer for this reason and what he found out was that it was the use of turmeric that was keeping leukemia on tabs. He has shown that from his studies that turmeric has the ability to irreversibly cease the multiplication of abnormal white blood cells that cause leukemia, in the bone marrow. The studies show that lifestyles like prenatal exposure to radiation, environmental pollutants like benzene and alkylating drugs contribute to the rise of childhood leukemia. Comprehensively the studies show that:

•   Turmeric inhibits chromosome damage caused by radiation.

•   Turmeric reduces the damage caused by carcinogenic chemicals that are created by the burning of carbon fuels like cigarette smoke.

- Turmeric prevents the creation of heterocyclic amines, harmful compounds that enter the body from processed foods.

Chapter #10: Cardiovascular Diseases

At this day and stage cholesterol is a word that is known to everyone; ask a 5 year old about it and he'll tell you about it. Cholesterol is not wholly bad but that's a whole other story. The thing one should know is that it is oxidized cholesterol that damages the blood vessels; it deposits in the plaque that become the reason for a heart attack or a stroke. Prevention of the oxidation of cholesterol can aid in the reduction of heart diseases and atherosclerosis.

Turmeric has a cholesterol lowering effect and this effect, like so many others is also owed to curcumin. Curcumin is acts like a messaging molecule that directs genes in the liver cells to increase the production of messenger proteins. These messenger proteins control the creation of bad (LDL) cholesterol receptors. With the help of these receptors, liver cells are able to clear more bad (LDL) cholesterol from the system.

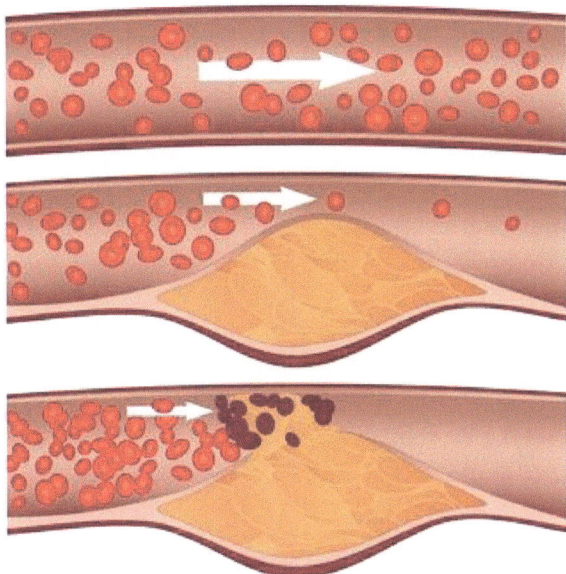

Cardiovascular diseases are not just related to cholesterol but there are other compounds in the background too; homocysteine is one of these compounds. It is an intermediate product of a cellular process that directly damages the walls of the blood vessels. High levels of homocysteine are a significant risk factor for atherosclerotic plaque build-up, blood vessel damage and heart disease. To keep the homocysteine levels from getting too high, vitamin B6 comes into play. A high intake of vitamin B6 reduces the risk of heart diseases by keeping the homocysteine to an optimized level.

A research was conducted on10 healthy volunteers, by the Indian Journal of Physiology and Pharmacology; they consumed 500mg of curcumin each day for 7 days. After 7 days it was found out that oxidized cholesterol in their blood dropped by 33% while the level of their good cholesterol increased by 29%.

Chapter # 11: Alzheimer's disease

Increasing evidence is suggesting that turmeric can help in fighting off neurodegenerative diseases like Alzheimer's. Alzheimer's disease is caused by protein fragment, amyloid-B that builds-up in the brain causing inflammation, oxidative stress and plaque formation between nerve cells.

How are plaques formed exactly? Firstly, amyloid is a term used for protein fragments normally found in the body. Amyloid-B is a fragment stripped from another protein called amyloid-PP. In a normal & healthy brain, amyloid-PP is broken and eliminated, however in patients of Alzheimer's, these fragments build-up and form hard, insoluble plaques. Moreover, in a healthy brain immune cells called macrophages are responsible for destroying abnormalities like amyloid-B but these immunities are rendered useless in Alzheimer's patients.

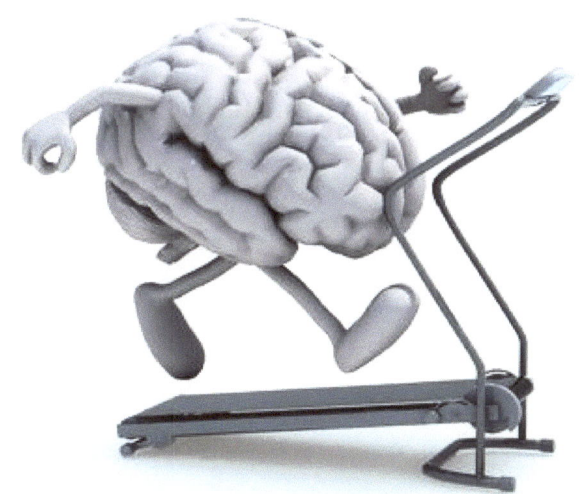

Researchers at UCLA conducted test tube studies that showed that curcumin reduced the build-up of amyloid-B and dissolved amyloid fibrils much more effectively than anti-inflammatory drugs like ibuprofen. Curcumin achieves this by binding to amyloid-B; once bound, these fragments can no longer clump and form plaques. And when it comes to revitalizing the immunity system, another variant of curcumin comes to play: bisdemethoxycurcumin. This chemical helps boost the activity of the immune system and macrophage levels. Dr. Milan Fiala and Dr. John Cashman conducted experiments on blood samples of Alzheimer's patients which concluded that bisdemethoxycurcumin increased the number of macrophages and promoted the clearance of amyloid-B in the brain.

Another layer of protection against Alzheimer's is provided by curcumin in the form of its anti-oxidant properties. Curcumin does so, by tapping a gene that orders the production of natural anti-oxidants in the brain. A study published in the Italian Journal of Biochemistry stated the role of curcumin in the induction of a pathway, heme oxygenase whose output is an anti-oxidant called bilirubin. The anti-oxidant prevents free radical injury to the brain; the same injury that is believed to be a major contributor for aging and cognitive diseases, one of which is Alzheimer.

Chapter # 12: Cancer

When it comes to cancer prevention, research on how turmeric does so is in very early stages and the current tests are only limited to lab or rodents. One such test has proved that due to its anti-oxidant properties, turmeric can prevent DNA mutations. Free radicals are responsible for DNA mutations that result in cell abnormalities during cell-replication; these abnormalities then become a major contributor of cancerous cells. By suppressing these free radicals, turmeric achieves the first layer of protection against cancerous cells.

Epidemiological studies have related the use of turmeric to lower rates of prostate, breast and colon cancer. Lab experiments have shown that curcumin can prevent the formation of tumors by interfering with several pathways known for their aid in the growth and spread of cancerous cells. Researchers at the University of Texas have carried out experiments on lab mice and concluded that turmeric can slow the spread of cancer in an already cancerous environment.

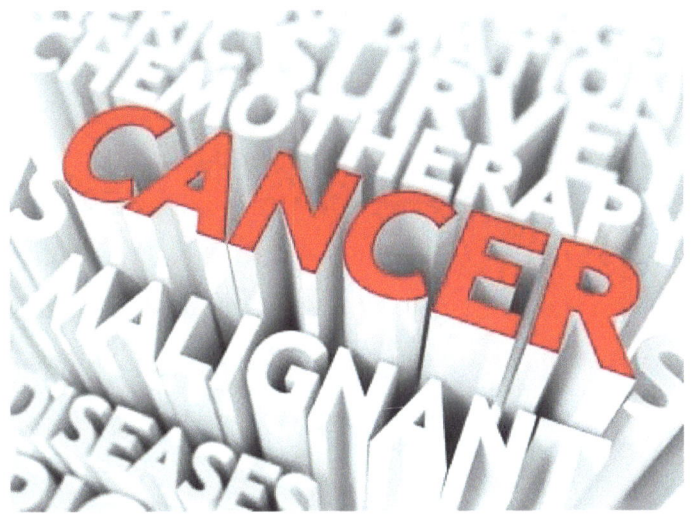

In their study published in 2005 in the paper Biochemical Pharmacology, cancerous breast cells were extracted from humans and injected into mice; the resulting tumors were removed, thus simulating a mastectomy. The mice were divided into 4 groups with:

- The first group receiving no further treatment.

- The second group receiving treatment with paclitaxel, a cancer drug.

- The third group receiving treatment with curcumin.

- The fourth group receiving treatment with both paclitaxel and curcumin.

After five weeks, 50% of the mice on curcumin and 22% on both paclitaxel & curcumin had indication of the breast cancer spreading to the lungs, while 75% of the mice that were on paclitaxel alone had developed tumors in the lung; 95% of the mice on no medication had developed lung cancer.

So how did curcumin aid the drug in suppressing the cancer from spreading? The lead researcher, Bharat Aggarwal stated that curcumin acted against transcription factors that regulate genes, needed for tumors to form. Inhibiting these factors down meant that genes that caused the growth of cancerous cells were effectively shut down.

In a lab study of non-Hodgkin lymphoma human cells, also published in Biochemical Pharmacology; researchers at the University of Texas showed that curcumin suppressed the initiation of a chain reaction that led to the promotion of cancerous cell growth. A regulatory molecule NF-kappaB signals the genes to produce a string of inflammatory molecules TNF, IL-6 and COX-2 that cause cancer cells to multiply. Curcumin stops this regulatory molecule thus, saving the body from a long list of troubles caused by the inflammatory molecules.

Turmeric and Onions team up against Colon Cancer

A research published in the 2006 issue of Clinical Gastroenterology and Hematology concluded that curcumin found in turmeric and quercitin, an anti-oxidant compound in onions can reduce the size as well as number of precancerous abnormalities in the intestinal tracts of humans. Five patients with an inherited case of precancerous tissue abnormalities in the lower bowel region were given regular doses of quercitin and curcumin over a period of six months. After six months the numbers of tissue abnormalities dropped by 60.4% while their size dropped by 50.9%.

These abnormalities found in the lower bowel are known as *familial adenomatous polyposis* or FAP. As the name suggests, FAP runs in families and involves the development of hundreds of tissues that eventually become fully cancerous cells. Lead researcher Francis M. Giariello at the Gastroenterology division at John Hopkins states that in recent times anti-inflammatory drugs such as ibuprofen and aspirin have been used to treat these conditions but the idea is being discouraged due to their serious side effects that include gastrointestinal bleedings and ulcerations.

Observational studies at a macro level have shown that societies that consume large amounts of turmeric rich foods have lower cases of intestinal problems such as colon cancer. Similarly, quercitin that is present mainly in onions and green tea has been found to subdue the growth of cancerous cells in humans.

Chapter # 13: A Super Spice

Till this day science has confirmed that turmeric is as good as 14 drugs. These drugs include:

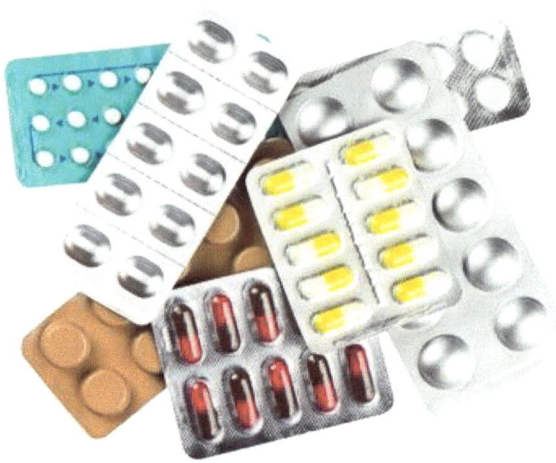

- **Lipitor/Atorvastatin (Medication for cholesterol):**

A 2008 study in the journal *Drugs in R&D* showed that a preparation of curcumin from turmeric worked similarly to the drug atorvastatin on improving the pathology of blood vessels that are associated with reductions in inflammation and oxidative stress.

- **Corticosteroid (steroid medications):**

Phytotherapy Research, a journal published in 1999 stated that curcumin compared favorably to steroids in the management of an inflammatory eye disease known as anterior uveitis. Also, curcumin had the medicinal worth of a drug, Corticosteroid that protects the lungs from transplantation injury.

- **Prozac/Fluoxetine & Imipramine (anti-depressants):**

A 2011 study in the journal, *Acta Poloniae Pharmaceutica*, that curcumin was effective in replicating the behavior of the body when treated with the drugs stated above in order to combat depressive behavior.

- **Aspirin (blood thinner):**

Study on effects of aspirin was conducted all the way back in 1986 and was published in Arzneimittelforschung. It was revealed that curcumin not only worked exactly like aspirin but also had an anti-platelet effect that indicated value for those who were liable to vascular diseases.

- **Anti-inflammatory drugs:**

A study published in *Oncogene* found that curcumin worked favorably with respect to anti-inflammatory drugs like ibuprofen, aspirin, sulindac, naproxen, phenylbutazone, indomethacin, dexamethasone, diclofenac, tamoxifen and celecoxib.

- **Oxaliplatin (Chemotherapy drug):**

The *International Journal of Cancer* reported that curcumin had similar effects to the anti-proliferative agent in colon, oxaliplatin.

- **Metformin (Diabetes drug):**

A study published in *Biochemistry and Biophysical Research Community* explored the possibility of curcumin treating diabetes. It was found out that curcumin was 500 – 100,000 times more potent in activating an enzyme that increases glucose uptake, when compared to metformin.

Conclusion

Everything you need to know about turmeric has been given in the book, from its history to its recipes, its medicinal worth and household use. This spice has innumerable benefits and if one can incorporate it in his/her daily routine, it can do wonders. Since it has no serious, life-threatening side-effect it can be consumed with no worries and as a matter of fact can make a lot of foods more lively and delicious.

So keep turmeric close to yourself and lead a healthy life.

Enjoy!

Author Bio

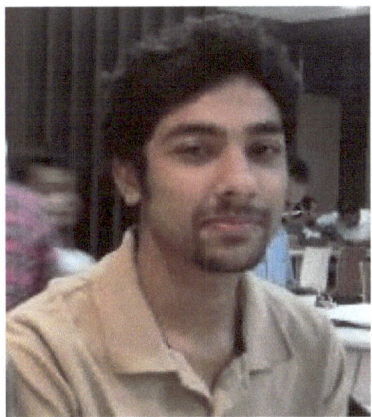

Muhammad Usman is a distinguished medical graduate of Allama iqbal medical college (AIMC). He is a professional writer who has been in the field for more than 4 years. During this time he has produced 10,000+ articles, blogs and eBooks on various niches related to diseases, health, fitness, nutrition and well-being. He is a regular contributor to several journals related to medicine and surgery. He is the editor of several journals and newspapers.

Check out some of the other JD-Biz Publishing books

Gardening Series on Amazon

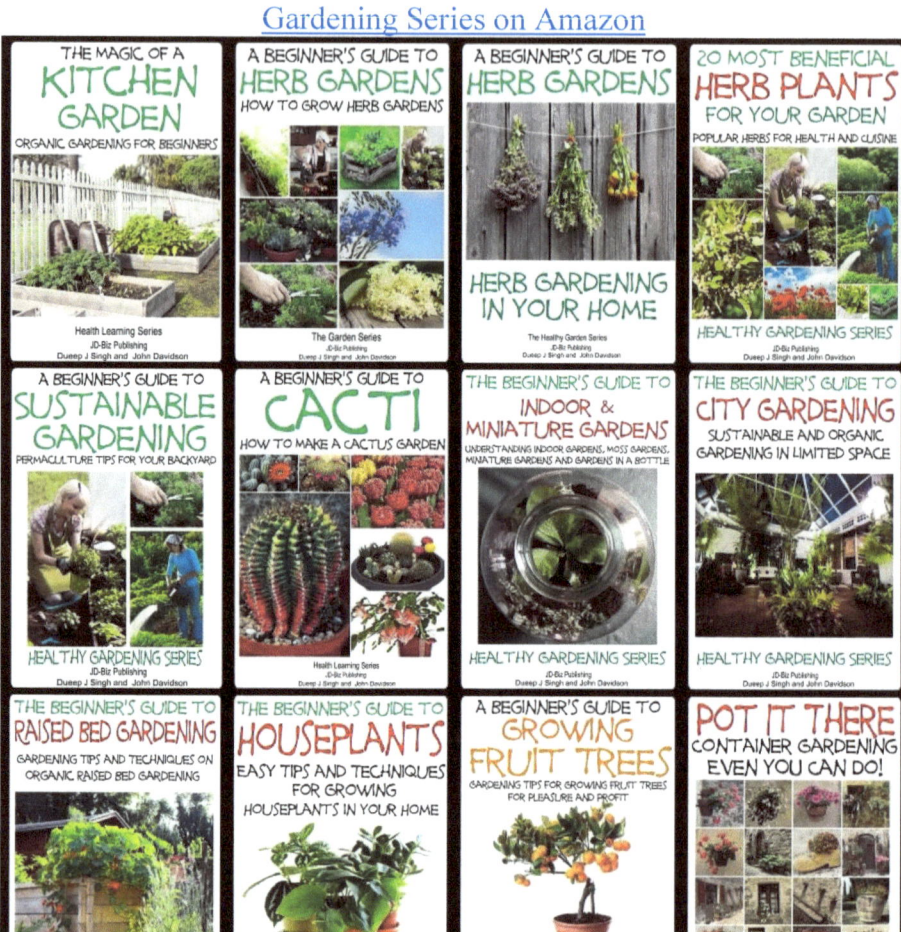

Download Free Books!

http://MendonCottageBooks.com

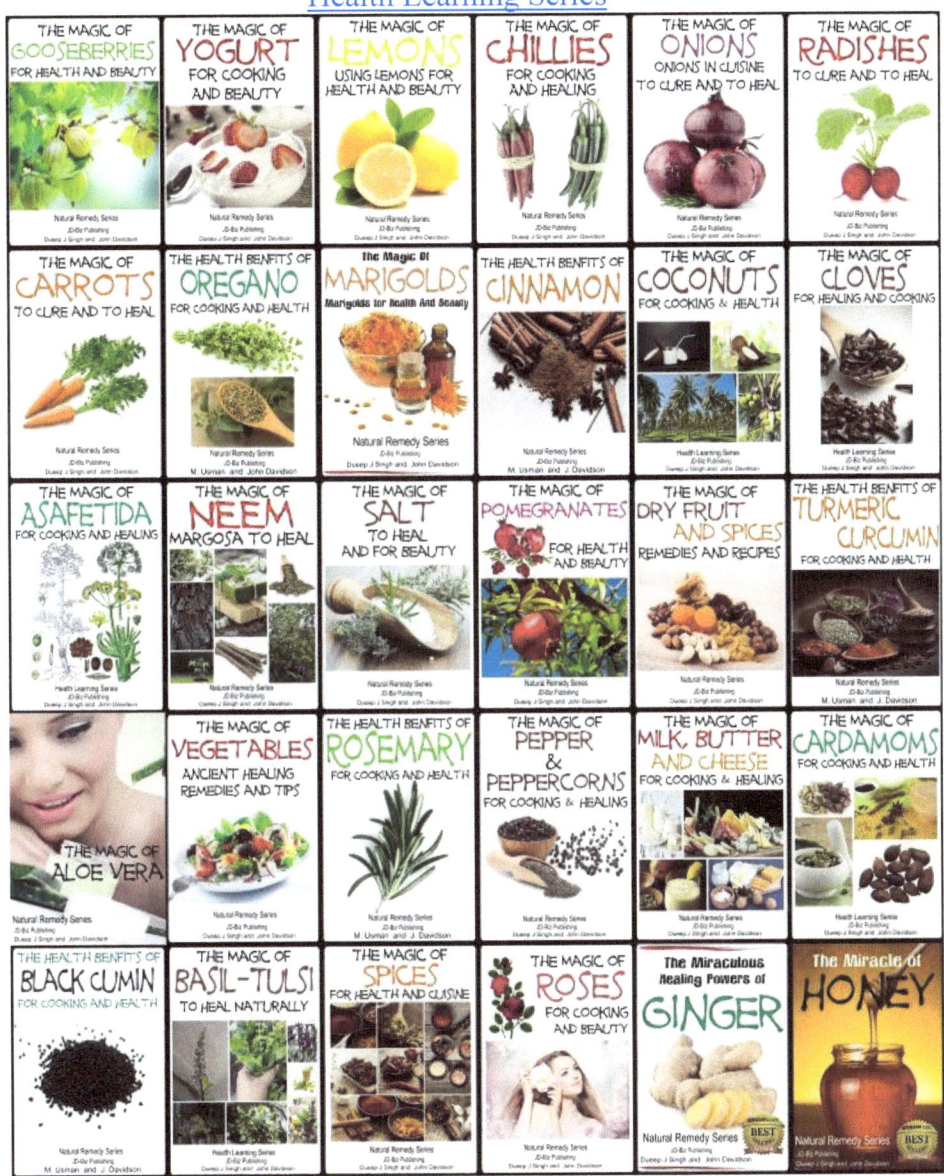

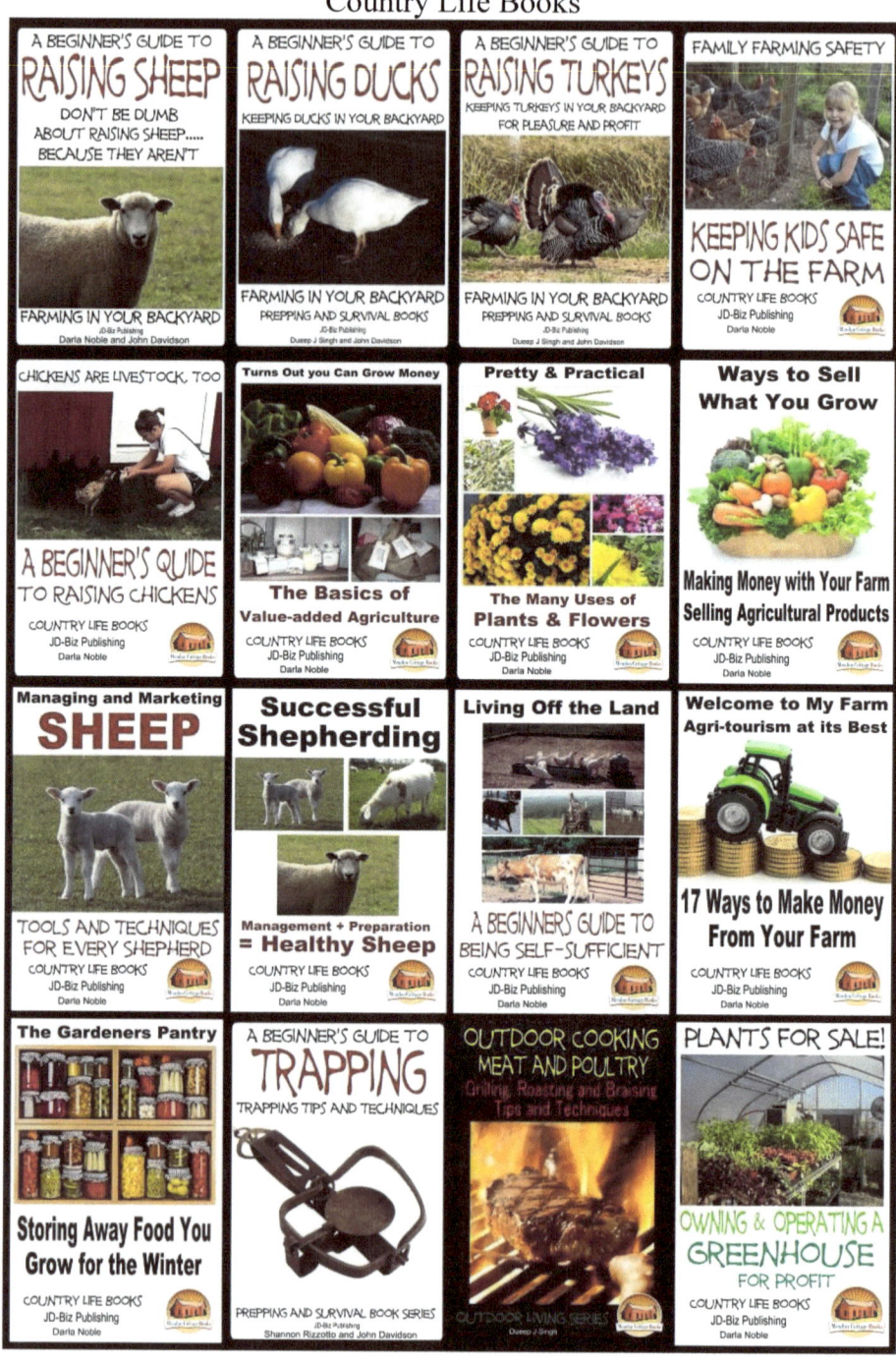

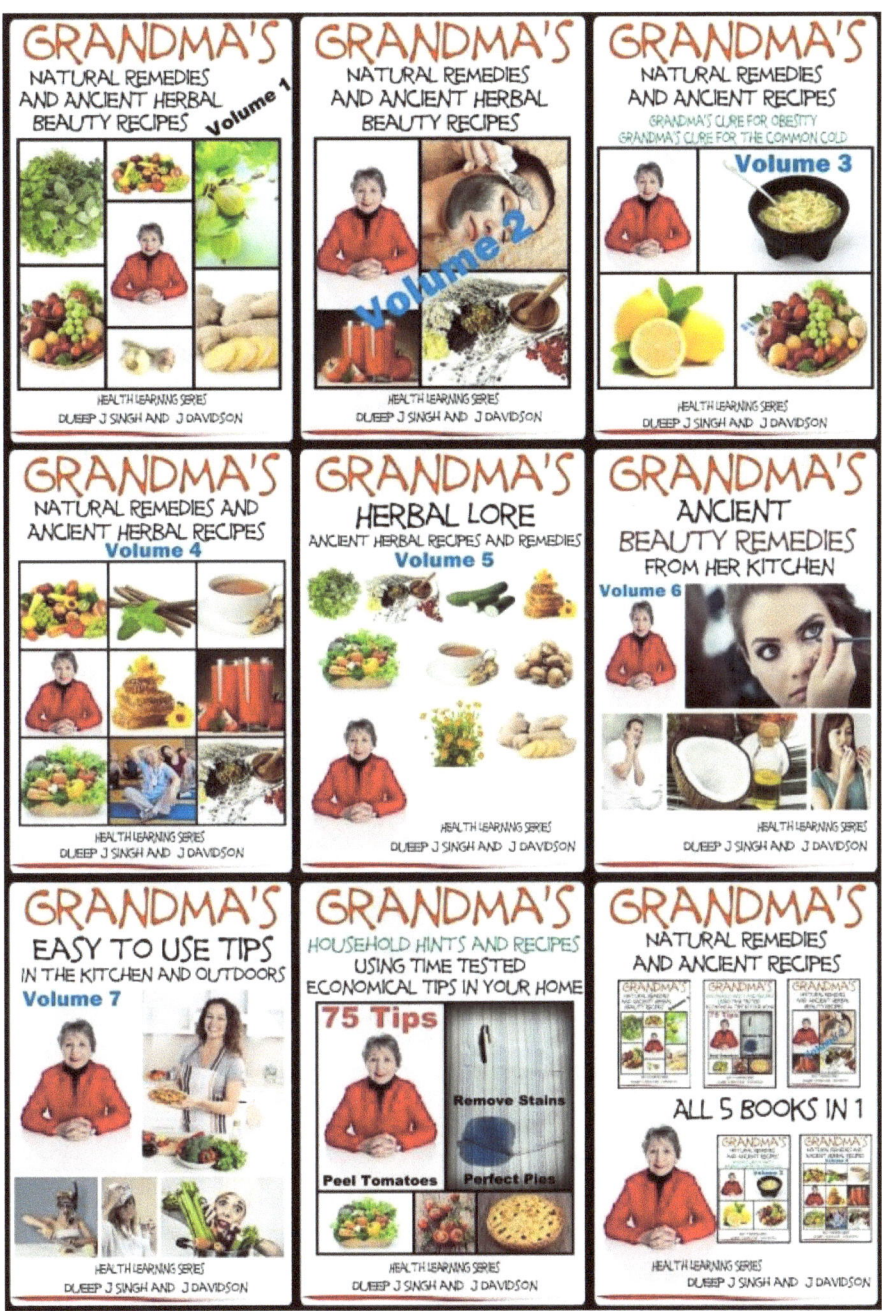

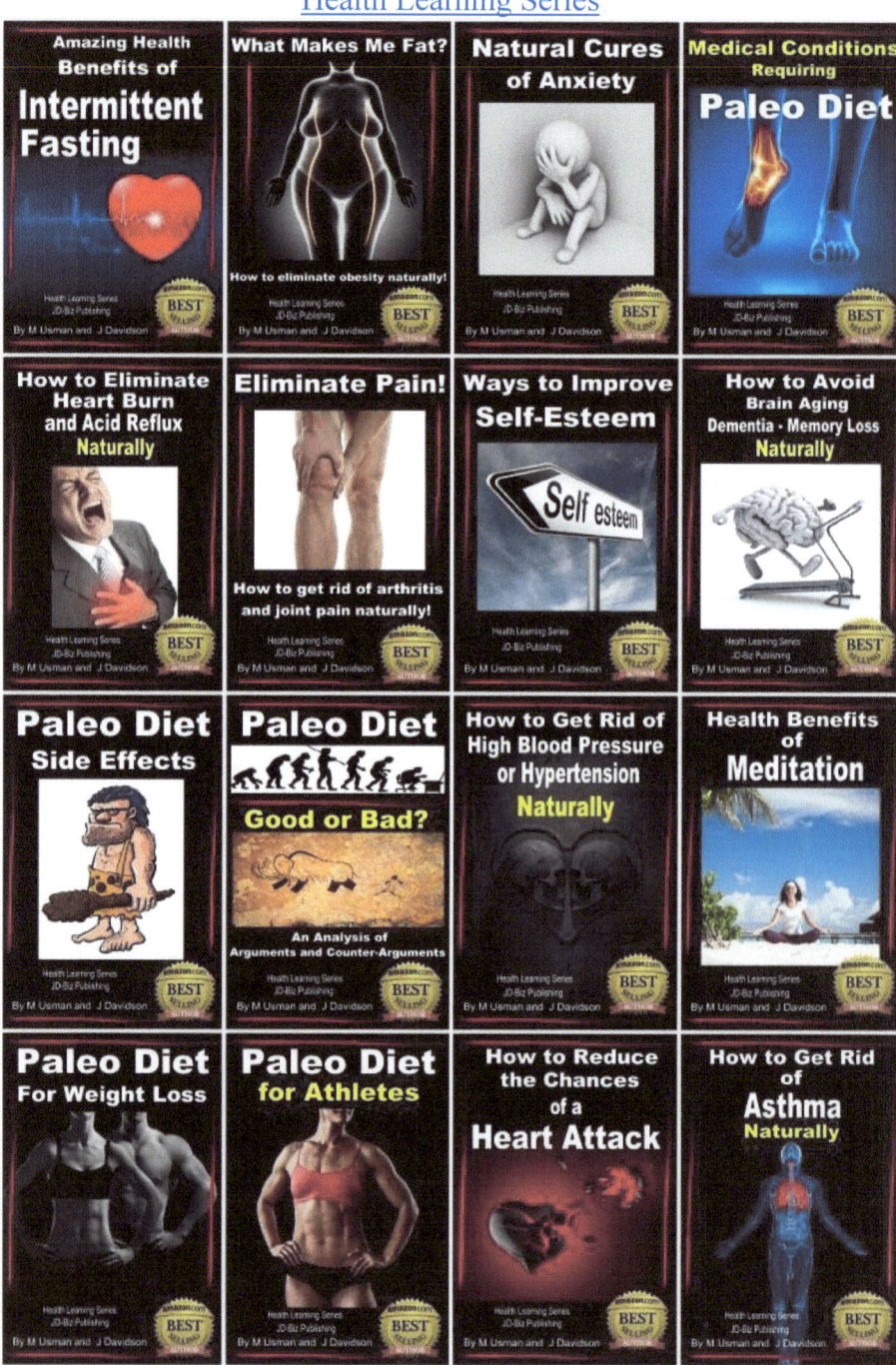

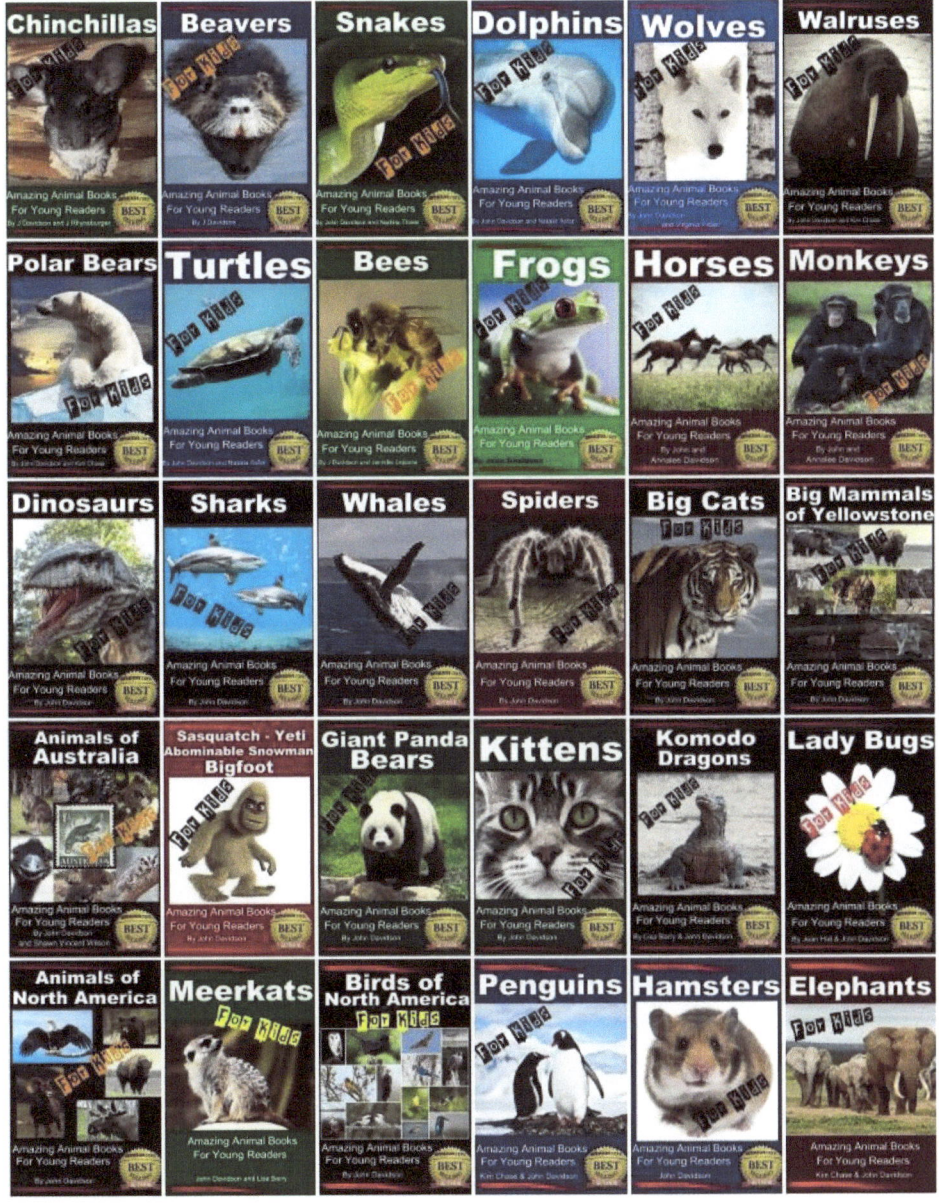

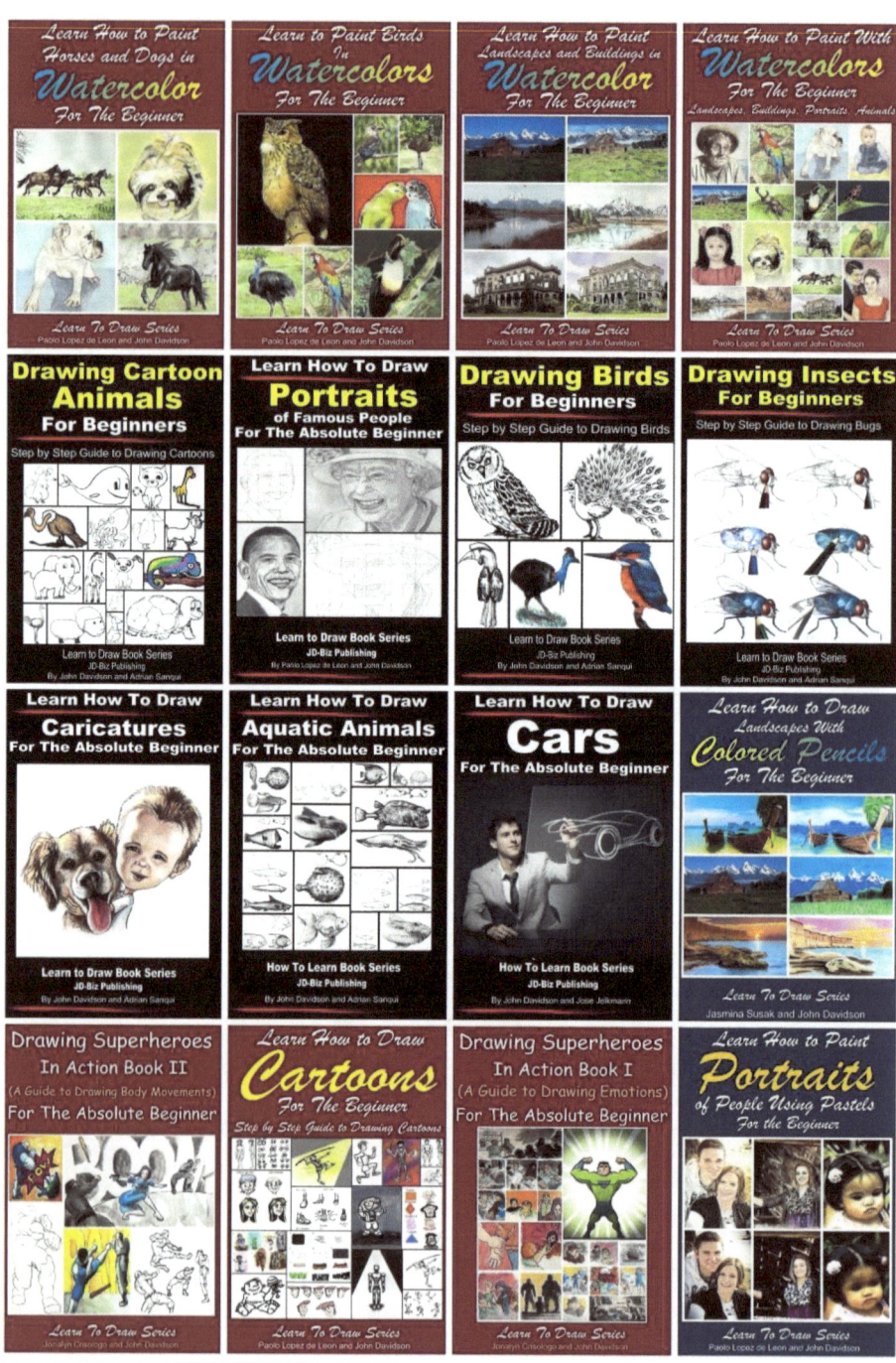

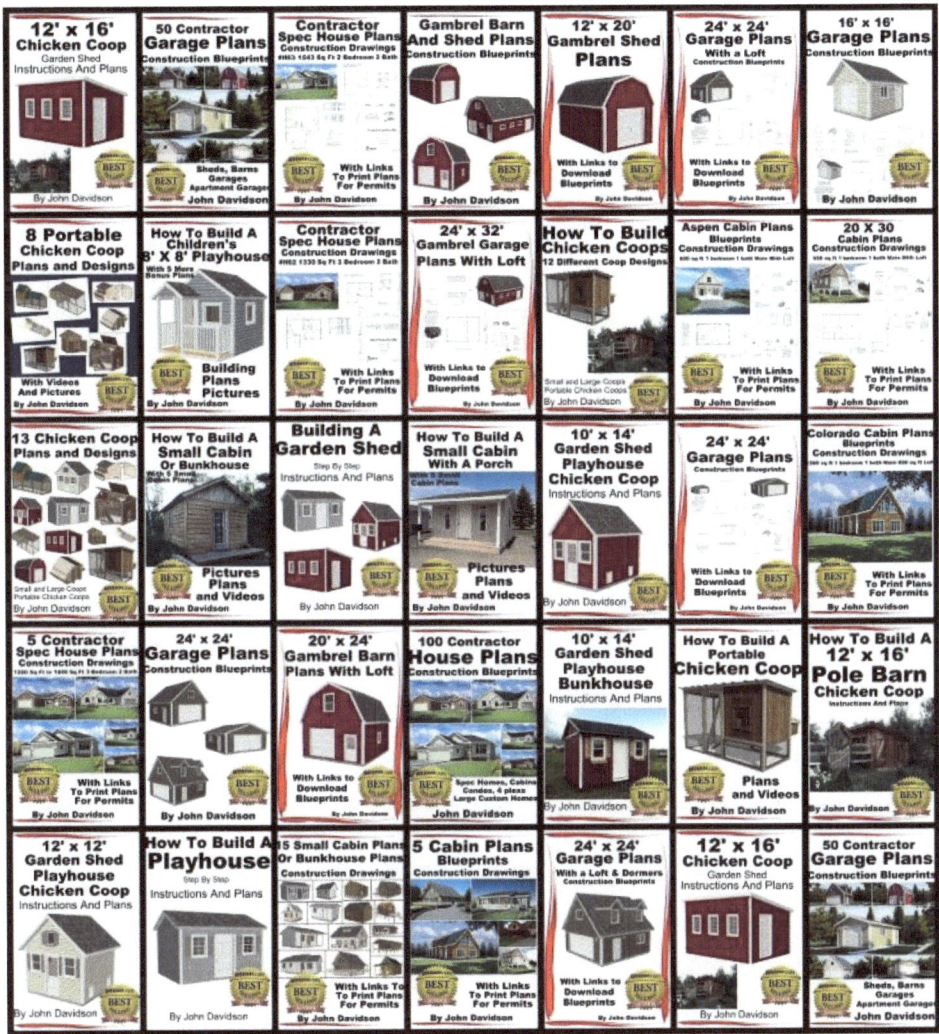

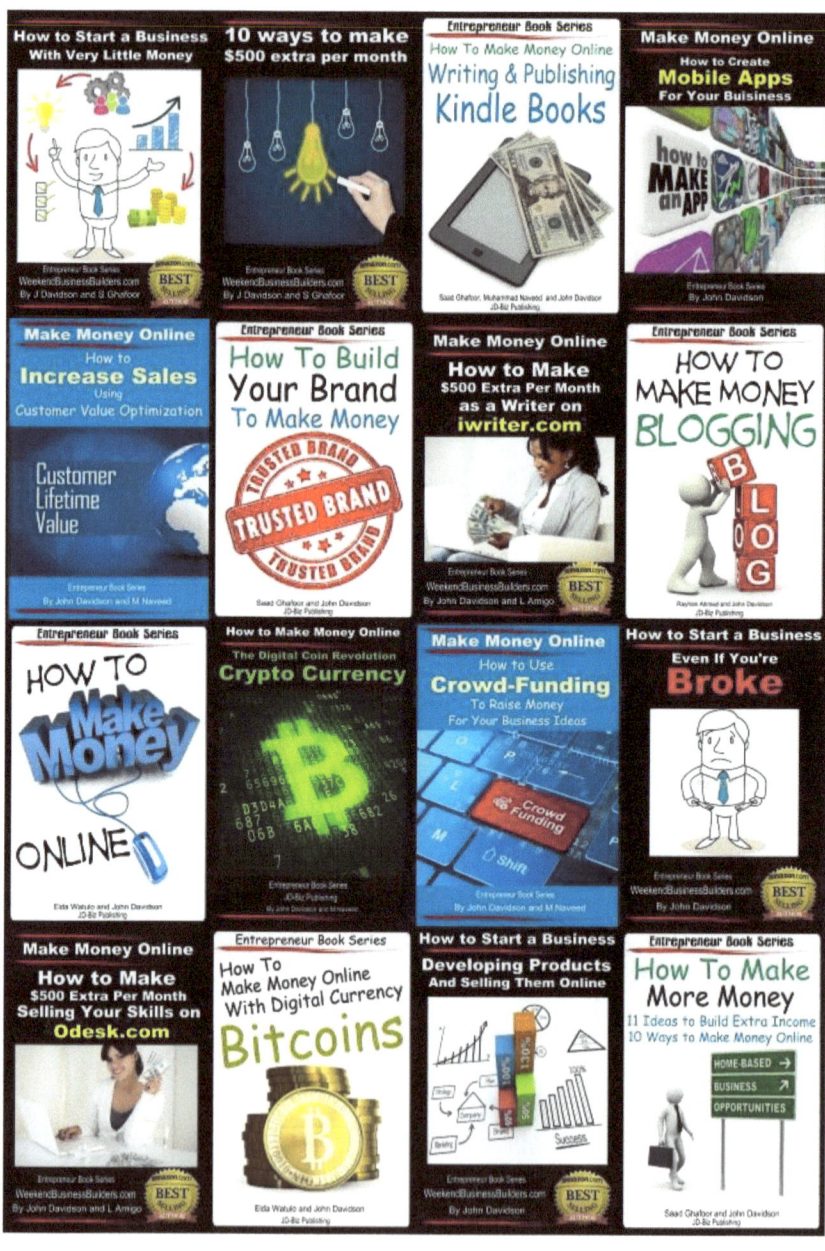

Our books are available at

1. Amazon.com
2. Barnes and Noble
3. Itunes
4. Kobo
5. Smashwords
6. Google Play Books

Download Free Books!

http://MendonCottageBooks.com

Publisher

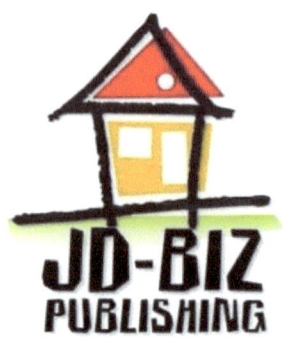

JD-Biz Corp

P O Box 374

Mendon, Utah 84325

http://www.jd-biz.com/

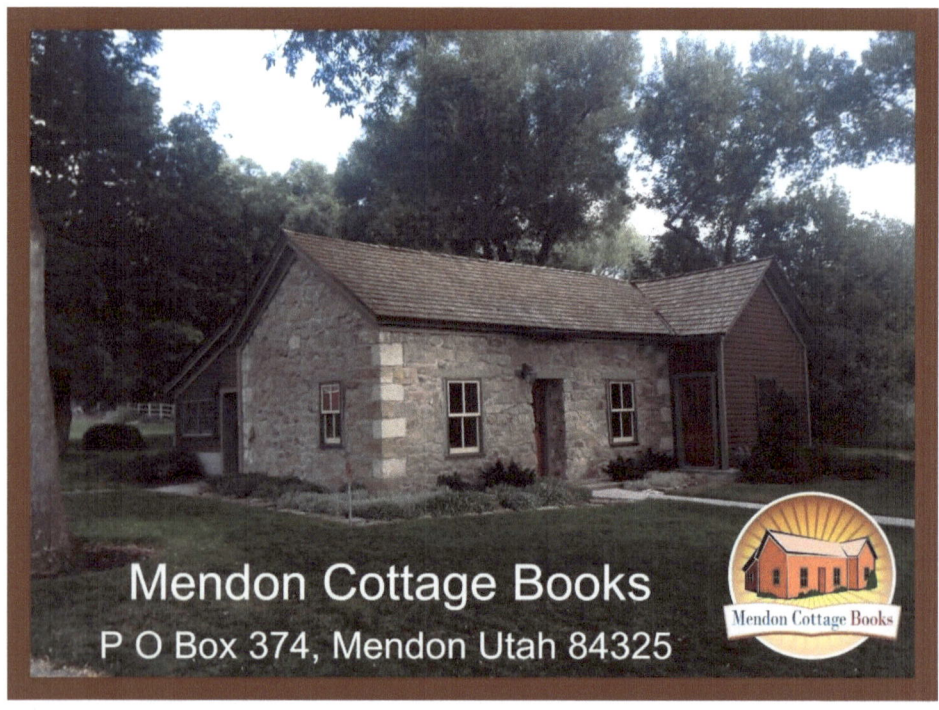